What Do We Know about Asthma?

Diagnosing and Treating Asthmatic Conditions

By: James M. Lowrance © 2011

To the many dedicated medical researchers and doctors who are accomplishing great things in the area of increased education and improved treatments for millions of asthma sufferers.

TABLE OF CONTENTS:

What Do We Know about Asthma?

INTRODUCTION:

Some Statistics including those by the Centers for Disease Control (CDC) state that up to 25-million Americans suffer from asthma. That's approximately I in every 12 people or about 8.2 percent of the US population. Asthma is more common in women than in men and is also more common among African Americans and Hispanics than in Caucasians.

Approximately 3,000 asthma deaths occur in the US each year. It is believed that undiagnosed asthma in a significantly large percent of sufferers in years past was due to less-adequate diagnosing of the disease. Better education on the types of asthma, its causes and related conditions (i.e. Chronic Bronchitis, Emphysema and COPD) is helping to detect more cases earlier, so that treatments can slow progression and improve the symptoms of these common respiratory diseases.

As a fellow asthma sufferer and patient advocate, it is my sincere hope that this book helps to educate its readers on this very important medical subject.
-*Jim Lowrance*

What Do We Know about Asthma?

CHAPTER ONE

My Personal Experience with Adult-Onset Asthma

Breathing is regulated by the involuntary nervous system but is something that we also consciously contribute-to and are aware of but that we often take for granted.

I slowly developed asthma as an adult in my mid-40s that is now in the "moderate-persistent" category. I only occasionally have to use an albuterol rescue inhaler with flares. My case of asthma may also have aspects of "upper airway resistance" involved because when I lay flat on my back (supine), I immediately feel some tightness in my lungs. When the upper airway is affected, this can be due to sinusitis, post nasal drip and esophageal digestive problems. This is however not uncommon with typical asthma, especially in those who also have GERD (Gastro Esophageal Reflux Disease) as I do. It naturally concerned me when these symptoms first manifested and I wanted to be assured by my MD, that there was no cardiac involvement (heart enlargement) in my asthma symptoms.

What Do We Know about Asthma?

I had her to order me a "BNP" blood test or "B-type Natriuretic Peptide" (when not abbreviated), which is very accurate for detecting congestive heart failure, even at the mildest levels. My lab result was "4" and I was very happy to see that result because elevated readings of 100 and above can indicate varied degrees of heart failure, which is always characterized by degrees of heart-enlargement.

BNP results that are between 300 to 600 represent moderate heart enlargement/failure and those at 900 and above represent severe cases of heart failure. Most people with asthma do not have Chronic Heart Failure (CHF – also called "Congestive Heart Failure") but if a person has risk factors for the condition, such as prolonged, chronic, untreated hypertension, heart valve problems, previous heart attacks and/or blockage in cardiac arteries or they are elderly, ruling out this potential cause of asthma may be important.

My GERD and anxiety (the anxiety being largely due to phases of mild hyperthyroidism from autoimmune thyroiditis) can be precipitating factors in my adult-onset case of asthma.

What Do We Know about Asthma?

I do have actual asthma and not simply the perception of restricted breathing or so-called "psychosomatic asthma" because I experience times of needing to clear mucous from my throat/lungs that forms in them at times and I experience cough and cough-sensations when taking in deep breaths or exhaling forcefully – such as with nose-blowing. I had asthma as a child as well but it stopped manifesting for many years and returned in my 40s, which is referred to as "adult onset asthma".

At night I sometimes hear some wheezing in my lungs, which is characteristic of asthma but also some clicking sounds with both the inhale and exhale of each breath when it is flaring. These sounds come from my lungs, not from my throat and there will be two or three of these faint clicks with each breath.

You might call it "crackling" but it isn't so prominent that I can feel it as some patients who experience this can. I can hear mine when it's quiet at night during bedtime hours when I am lying awake, especially during early morning hours.

What Do We Know about Asthma?

I bought a "peak flow meter" (PFM) - an Access Brand full-range one from Wal-Mart, made by Respironics Company. This is a device designed to measure the strength of the lungs at a given time and the amount of air the lungs are capable of holding. The price for one of these meters is cost-effective, considering its purpose in gauging changes in asthma severity. My meter cost less than $25.00 and it did not require a prescription from my doctor to be purchased. If an asthma patient suspects that an episode of worsening symptoms is eminent, a PFM can confirm the suspicion if an established personal best reading of lung function drops below 25%. A patient can then prepare for the asthma flare or possibly prevent much of its impact by using their rescue inhaler or by increasing their asthma medication dose, as directed by their doctor.

In some cases, asthma not only causes periods of lung weakness due to constricted and/or swollen breathing passages but also "hyperinflation" of them. This means it can be difficult to dispel all of the air inside of the lungs, before inhaling each new breath and it can also be difficult to take deep breaths to fully inflate the lungs.

What Do We Know about Asthma?

My PFM readings are usually very good, my best being about "800" and higher, which is above normal values for my age and height (approximately 600 is my predicted PFM normal value).I also had a chest/lung x-ray ordered by my MD (two views) and my lung tissue appears to be healthy and my heart size is normal, with no acute or chronic cardiopulmonary findings.

I've had the acid reflux disease for many years and I am moderately overweight. Within months of my adult asthma fully manifesting, I had several episodes of choking on stomach acid in bed at night, which made me wheeze and hyperventilate afterward.

Medical studies have shown that as many as 75% of asthma patients have GERD and that this disease of chronic acid reflux is a direct cause of asthma in some people.

Vitamin E and D deficiency are also contributors to asthma as well according to some medical research studies (possibly direct causes) and I have been diagnosed with both of these vitamin deficiencies, now being treated.

What Do We Know about Asthma?

Still, all-in-all my asthma is mild to moderate but usually persistent. I have never experienced any severe episodes and certainly none that have been life-threatening as some asthmatic patients experience and who are sometimes hospitalized in severe cases or when significant flares occur.

CHAPTER TWO

Simplified Descriptions of Asthma and Treatments

Asthma is an inflammatory disease of the lung passages (bronchial tubes), in which they begin to narrow and produce a thick, sticky mucous that causes wheezing and coughing, especially after exercise. Many asthma patients have worse symptoms at night and early morning and some have more difficulty breathing in the supine position (when lying down flat on their backs), especially if they are carrying extra weight around the midsection of the body.

Triggers for asthma can include things such as airborne allergens (i.e. pet dander, dust, pollen or chemicals), food allergies and air pollutions (i.e. smog, cigarette smoke and some chemical aerosol sprays) and obesity. For many asthma sufferers, physical exertion, especially aerobic types of exercise can serve as a trigger for episodes or "flares" as they are also called. In some patients, exercise alone can be the only identifiable asthma trigger.

What Do We Know about Asthma?

The vast majority of asthma cases are caused by allergies to things being inhaled from the air when taking-in oxygen. A more rare cause of asthma, is congestive heart failure (also referred to as "cardiac asthma"), in which a person with heart disease develops an enlarged heart, causing large amounts of fluid to build in the lungs, due to release of a hormone by the kidneys (BNP – "B-Type Natriuretic Peptide"), in response to stretching of the heart muscle. This type of asthma however is more common in heart disease patients and in the elderly and in people with serious heart defects and represents a very small percent of cases, when compared to the much more common allergic type asthma.

In people who already have asthma, stress, nervousness and anxiety can potentially trigger or worsen asthma symptoms as can things like acid reflux disease (GERD). Both asthma and GERD have potential to cause anxiety symptoms and chronic worry as well but qualified doctors can suggest something to help in these areas as well if asthma patients find difficulty in coping with either of these aggravating problems via lifestyle changes and or therapies.

There are self-help and psychiatric therapies, such as "Cognitive Behavioral Therapy" (CBT) that can help one deal with negative emotions resulting from asthma, including depression, or other co morbid physical illnesses (i.e. stress-related digestive disorders).

I personally used such coping methods when I was dealing with symptoms of autoimmune thyroid disease and associated health problems, which included anxiety symptoms and I found them to be very effective in reducing stress and emotional symptoms.

Can Asthma be Cured?

Asthma treatments are designed to control symptoms. Fast-acting inhalers (also called "rescue inhalers"), contain medications called "beta-agonists" and "bronchodilators", that relax the muscles surrounding the breathing passages and that help to open them, by reducing swelling that affects them. These also help mucous that forms in the lungs to be pushed out of them as the patient coughs.

What Do We Know about Asthma?

Rescue inhaler drugs that are in this category include the following:

• albuterol
• levalbuterol
• metaproterenol sulfate
• pirbuterol
• terbutaline

Long-term asthma control medications that may be prescribed may include the following:

• Corticosteroids (steroid anti-inflammatory)
• Leukotriene modifiers (non-steroid)
• Xolair injections (to help control allergies)
• Theophylline (for nighttime symptoms)
• Mast cell stabilizers (to control histamine)

While we can consciously change our breathing patterns, it is also an involuntary bodily function regulated by the nervous system (i.e. while we sleep). There is no cure for asthma, which can negatively affect the flow of breathing but it is usually a lifelong disease. Some asthma patients do however see the condition vary in severity, with months at a time not manifesting with flares or significant symptoms.

What Do We Know about Asthma?

Some asthmatics experience symptoms more-so in cold or hot months of the year or during those months when airborne allergens are at the highest (i.e. mold and pollen). Pets and household chemicals can also trigger asthma flares as previously mentioned. Controlling these type substances in the home and ridding the home of them when possible, can diminish asthma symptoms. Research studies have shown that up to 75% of people with asthma have acid reflux disease as well and they have well-established it as both an aggravator of asthma, as well as a direct cause of it. (Recommendations for controlling GERD will be addressed in a future chapter.)

Some studies state that GERD is more suspected as a direct cause of asthma, in adult-onset cases. I personally saw my adult-onset asthma manifest after several months of worsening acid reflux. On several occasions I awoke at night choking on stomach acid as previously mentioned, which burned my throat and caused my lungs to tighten and wheeze afterward. This was occurring despite my taking Prilosec, the prescription-strength over-the-counter acid blocker drug (also referred to as a "proton pump inhibitor").

What Do We Know about Asthma?

I feel I was having mild asthma for years previous, I just didn't recognize it as such. Asthma can also worsen bronchial infections resulting from colds or allergy flares.

A qualified doctor can rule-out other less common causes of asthma with chest x-rays and other tests that gauge lung strength and function. These will also rule out heart-involvement which is rare, especially if one hasn't experienced a heart attack or heart valve problems and if one is not elderly. If a person smokes, chronic bronchitis can be present as well and can co-exist with asthma (smoking and second-hand smoke can be detrimental to asthma patients). Chest x-rays can also detect tumors in the lungs that cause asthma type symptoms such as those found in cases of a disease called "sarcoidosis" and "pulmonary embolisms" (blood clots).

To repeat, there is no cure for asthma but it can be well-controlled with treatments as previously described. Lung infections in asthmatic patients will resolve completely over time with treatments such as antibiotics but this usually means they are susceptible to them with colds and flu (resulting in bronchitis flares).

What Do We Know about Asthma?

I'm a layperson and not a medical professional however the information contained in these chapters, comes from years of extensive search and research on many reputable medical information sources.

What Do We Know about Asthma?

CHAPTER THREE

Risks in Asthma Patients for Developing Future COPD

I have autoimmune thyroid disease, in addition to asthma, as previously mentioned and I have seen medical studies regarding patients with autoimmunity of any kind (autoimmune thyroiditis being specifically mentioned) being at higher risk for developing Chronic Obstructive Pulmonary Disease (COPD) in later life. COPD is not actually one specific breathing problem, in-fact some sources I've frequented for researching the subject, also place typical asthma in the same category with COPD.

I've mentioned in past articles I have written, online, although hopefully each time it hasn't come across negatively judgmental toward some in the medical community, that with each medical issue I have researched for articles and books, I will find conflicting information regarding "risk factors" for particular diseases and even regarding best treatments for them.

Some sources seemingly lump all COPD cases into one category, to include asthma and some imply that it always leads to an eventual dramatic progression and that it is always irreversible. I would think that this would actually depend on the type of COPD one has (i.e. chronic bronchitis, types of asthma or emphysema). In regard to Peak Flow Meters used to monitor and even to sometimes diagnose respiratory disorders, most sources agree with the need for "Pulmonary Function Testing" PFT to definitively diagnose COPD (more sophisticated than PFM monitoring).

That certainly makes sense however some sources also say that both typical asthma and COPD are commonly misdiagnosed, even with the full-array of tests being ordered for diagnosis (including those conducted by pulmonary specialists). These type issues are frustrating and a bit disturbing but all we who have asthma can do as patients is to go through all of the available diagnostic processes, including follow-up monitoring of our individual cases and to follow any treatment plans recommended to us as a result by our doctors.

What Do We Know about Asthma?

Some medical information sources make statements on particular aspects of asthma and COPD cases but they leave out important details in them. It is not that I feel those types of articles can be perfect, with so many variables often being involved among the group-patient cases being studied. Sometimes however, I find that some key information is not being mentioned in some of these abstract research articles that are published online (this is certainly not true of all of them). This type of information is too important in my opinion, to not be given better detail for the sake of patients seeking information not being supplied to them by their doctors, due to their heavy schedules and lack of time to properly educate their patients.

Here for example, is what the U.S. National Institutes of Health page says in regard to Peak Flow Meters:

"The peak expiratory flow rate measures how fast a person can breathe out (exhale) air. It is one of many tests that measures how well the lungs are working.

What Do We Know about Asthma?

The test is commonly used to diagnose and monitor lung diseases such as:

Asthma
Chronic obstructive pulmonary disease (COPD)
Rejection after a lung transplant

Home monitoring can help determine whether treatments are working or detect when your condition is getting worse. "

What is doesn't mention is that peak flow rate alone doesn't provide an initial diagnosis. This is likely mentioned on some of their other pages.

Despite this, other medical research articles state that some doctors go no further with testing a patient if their peak flow reading is normal or above normal. This-too is somewhat understandable because peak flow is affected in COPD cases as well, even without co morbid asthma being present, when it reaches moderate and severe levels.

The Mayo Clinic site states that GERD may cause COPD in some people.

What Do We Know about Asthma?

They don't however, add any detail as to whether they mean that this can be the case with those who also smoke or who are elderly, etc... Other medical sites that are just as reputable if not more so than the Mayo Clinic, state that GERD has been found to exacerbate flares of COPD but that there are no studies that directly attribute it as a "cause" of COPD. Some sources out there state that typical asthma is also a disease of COPD (chronic lung obstruction); while others state that the differences are very distinct between asthma and COPD (i.e. asthma is reversible obstruction while COPD is not reversible).

This is yet another aspect of opposing views being expressed that causes confusion to patients who may search for online information regarding respiratory disorders. I think each of us has to let that perspective between these information sources balance in our own minds the best possible and to follow our prescribed treatments accordingly.

I have to admit that I can't imagine typical asthma not also being recognized as "obstructive" in nature.

What Do We Know about Asthma?

It may be that the "chronic" aspect that makes some of these sources differentiate between asthma and COPD, conveys the fact that there is ongoing, clearly identifiable lung damage in COPD, while asthma may reverse and in some cases actually go into remission for periods of time or even permanently. The search and research continues for all of us, including that being conducted by the medical research group professionals, who are working hard to find better treatments and possible cures. I'm personally thankful for their efforts, regardless of some of the conflicting information that currently exists out there regarding both asthma and COPD.

CHAPTER FOUR

Medical Research Statistics on the COPD – Asthma Connection

Medical research quote:

"In a 20-year, follow-up study published in "Chest Journal" (The American College of Chest Physicians), compared to non-asthmatics, patients who had asthma had a 10-times-higher risk for acquiring symptoms of chronic bronchitis, a 17-times-higher risk of receiving a diagnosis of emphysema, and a 12.5-times-higher risk of meeting criteria necessary to diagnose COPD. This was even after adjustments were made for smoking history and other potential confounders. So, although asthma and COPD are distinct entities, and have different physiological features and risk factors, having asthma is significantly associated with an increased risk for the development of COPD." (About.com – Asthma Guide)

A "17 times higher risk for COPD?" This is a huge number.

I know because I see medical statistics often and even a 4 times higher risk is significant. I did find slightly more information at the WebMD website, regarding these same statistics that I first found at the About.com Asthma Guide site but there is a great deal of detail still missing regarding the 3,099 adult patients who were studied. I then found the original medical study abstract and sure enough the statement in the original research article was there. It adds to the statement in regard to the very high risk of COPD in asthma patients, that "even after adjustments were made for smoking history and other potential confounders". This was in the abstract published for online viewing.

This statement, from my personal view gives the impression that they are saying that smoking was not a relevant issue in that particular study (I may be incorrect in this interpretation). The original online abstract also didn't include the wording that the WebMD article includes, saying that the risk of developing COPD in asthma patients is "later in life". It is unclear if this means when a person reaches senior-age years or if age makes no difference.

What Do We Know about Asthma?

There is however a study WebMD cites titled "Childhood Asthma Linked to Risk of COPD" and in this one, they state that the study showed that that risk for COPD was increased "32 times" in children with severe asthma, who developed COPD 50 years later in life (obviously in their 50s or 60s). There was however no mention of how many were current or previous smokers. That's an important detail that one would like to see included (No offense to WebMD. I appreciate their site and they were simply citing a research study).

I think these medical researchers are certainly doing their best in advancing knowledge and treatments for asthma and other respiratory problems and I'm thankful for them as previously mentioned. It is however, a bit frustrating, as also mentioned previously, to not see more specifics in the abstracts and even in the full documents published by medical entities. If they can go the extent of such studies involving 1,000s of patient-participants, I personally would love to see every possible detail included for best-possible perspective because "the devil is in the details" so-to-speak.

What Do We Know about Asthma?

Medical studies of these types can also be in varied degrees of contradiction with each other. For example, I have seen other studies state to-the-effect: "we do not believe asthma becomes COPD or that COPD becomes asthma". Medical researchers are human like the rest of us. They can make mistakes and disagree among each other, as with all areas of scientific research. Still, I'm proud to see the vast progress in so many areas and that they continue to whittle-away at these common diseases affecting humanity.

I would have also liked to have known the average ages of the respondents/participants in the study showing a 17-times risk of COPD in asthma patients. If for example the 3,099 "adults" studied, included anyone of adult age, such as ages 18, 21 or 25, did these younger folks also have these 10-fold, 12.5-fold and 17-fold chances of developing types of COPD? If age didn't matter a great deal, does this mean that folks even in childhood, whose asthma remains persistent throughout the years of their lives, also develop these more serious obstructive lung diseases within about 20 years? Some online information also varies widely between medical research groups, regarding asthma statistics.

What Do We Know about Asthma?

Some can be published during the same years but statistics of how many Americans suffer asthma can vary by 5 million from one information site to the next (i.e. 17-million asthma patients nationwide in the USA, versus 22-million - a significant variance).

Here's a quote from the Wkipedia page on asthma (they are not a medical cite but glean all their information from reputable medical sources):

"In 2005 in the United States asthma affected more than 22 million people including 6 million children." This information obviously means that far more adults suffer asthma than do children (over 3 and 1/2 times as many adults).

Some of the medical information websites I have searched however left me the impression that asthma is more common in children but this likely has to do with the "missing info" I've been referring to in reference to some information sources. That's why I always confirm any online information I search on medical subjects, with lots of different reputable sources.

What Do We Know about Asthma?

I highly recommend this be done by other laypersons looking for more information on their health disorders online.

When Medical Studies Conflict

It can be frustrating at times when studies or sets of medical information of any kind are diametrically opposed but in most cases it is simply a difference regarding specific factors.

I'll add one more example in concluding this chapter:

My own case of adult onset asthma in my late - 40s is almost certainly a direct cause of my GERD. I'm not a smoker and have no obvious allergies, although it's possible I have some food intolerances that act similar to allergens. I started searching on the subject of the "GERD and asthma connection" and it is very well established as not only a contributor but a "cause" of asthma. While doing the search I came across a Mayo Clinic page stating that GERD may also be a cause of COPD in some people.

What Do We Know about Asthma?

Quote: "GERD can make COPD worse and may even cause it in some people."
link:
http://www.mayoclinic.com/health/copd/DS00916/DSECTION=risk-factors

I decided to email a respiratory specializing hospital (National Jewish Health Center), asking them a question about peak flow meters and about GERD being a "cause" of COPD and they straightforwardly stated that it is not a cause of COPD but a well confirmed cause of asthma.

Here is a quote from that email they sent back in reply to me:

"There is a well know group of individuals for whom peak flow meters don't work. I am not worried about COPD since you have no smoking history. GERD does not cause COPD but is a well-known asthma trigger. I hope you are on medication for your asthma. I would not worry about the peak flow meter. Your physician should do spirometry or pulmonary function testing which is much more accurate. Good luck.

What Do We Know about Asthma?

Please feel free to email again with further questions."

So...here again, another contradictory bit of information, however, despite this, I truly appreciate both medical entities and I have benefited from their sources many times over. I will just continue to do the best I can in balancing all of the information I find on a given subject but I will also continue to stick to the best possible sources, including these I have named.

CHAPTER FIVE

Can Acid Reflux Disease Trigger the Development of Asthma?

My response that follows below was to someone who posted a comment to me on an online article I wrote, asking about the connection of their GERD to asthma symptoms they also developed after contracting a flu virus. ---

My reply:

"This is layperson, non-med pro opinion of course but one thing that comes to mind is that your years of GERD may have started some inflammation in your lungs but had not yet manifested as asthma. The flu virus may have been a trigger that brought the asthma to the surface that was in a sense dormant in your body. My own asthma manifested in me in my 40s but I could remember times past that I had mild indications of it. I in fact remember one particular asthma flare that occurred several years ago and I wondered at that time if an allergen of some type had triggered a solitary flare.

I now believe the asthma was there for quite some time, it just took a while for it to fully reveal itself. I believe adult asthma can have a slow onset. Severe cases of GERD should be evaluated by a Gastroenterologist.

Gastroenterologists specialize in the diagnosis and treatment of health disorders affecting the large and small intestines and esophageal disorders (affecting the esophagus). These would be conditions such as Irritable Bowel Syndrome, Crohn's disease, Ulcers, Gastro esophageal Reflux Disease (acid reflux), parasites, colon cancer (may also require an Oncologist) and other disorders of the digestive system.

Gastroenterology is the practice these doctors specialize-in by providing definitive diagnoses through tests such as upper and lowers G.I.s (Barium x-rays), colonoscopies and blood lab testing. Once they have diagnosed conditions present in patients, they give them the appropriate treatments needed, which may include drug therapies, specialized diets and/or surgeries to control symptoms or to resolve the underlying conditions."

What Do We Know about Asthma?

More on Acid Reflux and Lung Disorders

(GERD and Respiratory Illnesses)

Gastro Esophageal Reflux Disease (GERD) is a common cause of breathing problems, including bronchitis, asthma and pneumonia.

GERD can be a direct trigger for these pulmonary (lung) disorders or can worsen them in people with an already existing breathing problem. This occurs due to acid from the stomach, making its way into the windpipe and/or breathing tubes of the lungs. There are treatments available for the acid reflux that can lead to these respiratory problems.

What is GERD?

Gastro Esophageal Reflux Disease is a condition in which contents in the stomach, such as food, liquids and stomach-acid travel up into the esophagus causing a heartburn sensation. The esophagus is the tube that goes from the mouth down to the stomach and there is an upper valve that closes it off from the windpipe with swallowing (the sphincter) to prevent food from being inhaled.

What Causes GERD?

GERD can occur over time with consuming spicy and/or foods or with eating very large meals. It can be aggravated by eating too close to bedtime, in which the full stomach has not had time to fully digest its contents (indigestion).

It can also manifest more severely with excess weight in the mid-section, which adds pressure on the stomach, especially when lying flat on one's back.

The typical symptoms of GERD may include the following.

• heart burn

• sour stomach

• bitter flavor in the mouth

• mild chest pain

• an urge to swallow often

• a sensation of food moving upward into the throat

What Do We Know about Asthma?

How GERD Affects Breathing

While food may not make its way into the windpipe when acid reflux occurs, stomach acid may still irritate the upper portion of the esophagus and the opening of the windpipe. Over time, very small amounts of stomach acid will seep into the lungs, causing irritation of the breathing passages in the lungs (bronchial tubes). Some GERD sufferers can experience episodes of actually choking on stomach acid and/or food particles that make their way into the breathing tube.

Symptoms of a breathing problem can include the following.

• coughing

• wheezing

• popping or crackling sounds when breathing

• uncomfortable feeling in the chest (usually tightness)

• shortness of breath with mild exertion

Resulting Breathing Disorders

A common breathing problem that can result from GERD is bronchitis, which is a term simply meaning that the bronchial tubes have become irritated and inflamed which often causes them to become congested. Some cases of bronchitis first manifest with a dry cough (non-productive) and afterward, the lungs will begin to secrete mucous (phlegm) in an attempt to push out bacteria and inflammation. At this point, the cough becomes productive (or may start out productive). The phlegm will often remain as a clear-colored non-infectious type that clears-up over an approximate two week period.

In more severe cases of bronchitis, the phlegm may develop into a white, green or yellow color or have streaks of blood found in it, which can indicate developing pneumonia or chronic bronchitis (ongoing). These are more serious forms of infectious lung illness that can cause permanent lung damage and scarring and may contribute to COPD (Chronic Obstructive Pulmonary Disease). It can also become an emergency situation and can require hospitalization due to the extreme difficulty in breathing that can result.

What Do We Know about Asthma?

Asthma is also a common finding in GERD patients and this condition simply indicates that the bronchial tubes in the lungs are constricting, causing difficulty with breathing. Cases of asthma can be mild, moderate or severe. This constriction within the lungs in cases of GERD is the body's attempt to prevent more food particles or acid from entering into them. Sometimes bronchitis and asthma occur together, which is referred to as "bronchial asthma."

Stomach Acid from GERD Entering the Lungs

The following was a response I made to someone who posted a question to me, regarding what a person should do if they breathe stomach acid into their lungs:

"There's very little information available online as far as medical sources recommending what to do in the case of acid already entering the lungs (aspired). I too have experienced this, actually choking several times and feeling the acid coming back up from my lungs into my throat when coughing (very strong burning sensation).

What Do We Know about Asthma?

My suspicion however is that the body rids itself of the acid that travels to the lungs over time, which of course is foreign to them. The body likely does this by producing mucous, which will cause the stomach acid to be coughed up. This is also in-part how asthma symptoms result from acid reflux disease. The acid also likely causes an inflammatory reaction which asthma sources state is part of the reason breathing passages narrow and tighten, when reacting to asthma triggers.

I also found over time with my own asthma that I experienced "orthopnea" - more difficult to breathe lying flat on my back - supine. This concerned me greatly at first but I found medical information sources stating that orthopnea is common with GERD and some doctors speculate that the lungs begin to close when they sense the supine position to prevent more acid from entering into them and causing further damage.

I would suggest that if you feel acid go into your windpipe, that you should purposely induce a cough until you feel you've rid your lungs of it, as best possible. Medical sources also recommend elevating the head of your bed by six inches by placing books or bricks under it.

What Do We Know about Asthma?

Also taking an acid blocker drug such as Prilosec or Prevacid can help a great deal as well, as can as-needed antacid tablets such as Rolaids or TUMS. It is important to see your doctor when acid reflux is severe, meaning chronic and ongoing, rather than occasional or mild in occurrence."

More on Treatments for Acid Reflux

Research studies have shown that 75% of people with chronic cough from bronchitis and/or asthma will improve with treatment of co-morbid (co-occurring) GERD. Treatments may include over-the-counter antacids, prescription acid blocker medications (H2-blockers) and lifestyle changes.

Doctors will often recommend that patients lose excess weight and eat lighter meals that are not spicy. They may also recommend that GERD patients elevate the head of their beds a few inches as previously mentioned. This helps to keep acid from rising into the throat and eating evening meals no closer than three hours before bedtime can help with acid reflux problems as well.

Severe damage (erosion) of the esophagus can result in the need for surgical repair and some cases of GERD develop into a condition called "Barrett's Esophagus", a pre-cancerous condition that may require removal of a section of the esophagus.

While actual breathing disorders require separate treatments of their own, treating GERD can help to prevent these illnesses from developing and help patients to recover or improve from existing breathing disorders.

CHAPTER SIX

Understanding Congestive Heart Failure and Cardiac Asthma

(A Chronic but Treatable Condition)

Congestive Heart Failure (CHF) is more common in people ages 65 and older but can affect people at any age who have defects or damage to their heart muscles.

In most patients, CHF has a chronic course but can be reversed in some cases. Even when it remains chronic (ongoing) treatments can be administered to treat symptoms and to improve quality of life for CHF patients. In some cases, fluid may build in a patient's lungs and/or their heart may become enlarged but there are treatments to relieve symptoms caused by complications of CHF.

Symptoms of CHF

The symptoms can vary among individuals, but the ones that are typically experienced may include the following:

• shortness of breath ---

What Do We Know about Asthma?

- wheezing and coughing

- edema in the ankles or abdomen (swelling)

- fatigue

- heart enlargement

- exercise intolerance

- failure in other organs of the body (i.e. kidneys, liver and brain)

These symptoms occur due to a weakening of the heart muscle over time, which causes inadequate supply of blood circulation to the muscles and organs of the body. A resulting effect of diminished heart function out-put, includes a build-up of fluid around the heart and in the lungs, which also contributes to symptoms.

Causes of CHF

Conditions that cause heart arrhythmias and damage to the heart muscle can result in the development of CHF over time. If a person has a heart murmur or birth defect in the heart, for example, this can cause the condition to develop as they age and especially when they reach their senior-age years.

What Do We Know about Asthma?

Heart attacks can also contribute to the development of CHF due to the resulting damage in the heart muscle that causes less-adequate heart function as a person ages. As the heart muscle struggles to supply proper blood circulation output while it is in a damaged or inadequately functioning state, it will often become enlarged. This is its attempt to allow more blood-flow through the heart valves but is a serious development that can require emergency care.

Lifestyle Treatments for CHF

If the condition is mild to moderate and not causing significant symptoms, a treating doctor might simply prescribe lifestyle changes and intermittent short-term use of a diuretic medication (for fluid retention). These changes in lifestyle might include the following:

• losing excess weight in the body

• regular exercise at proper tolerance level

• a healthy diet

• reduced fluid intake

• removing sodium from the diet (salt – which results in fluid retention)

What Do We Know about Asthma?

This type of regimen would be monitored closely by regular follow ups with the patient, to see if the treatment is working or if prescription medications need to be added.

Prescription and Surgical Treatments

Prescribed medications for more severe cases might include beta-blocker drugs to control hypertension, cardiac glycosides to increase cardiac output and ACE Inhibitors to prevent renin released by the kidneys from converting into angiotensin II (a hormone that causes heart constriction).

Should CHF worsen despite prescribed treatments, these worst-case scenarios might require corrective surgery for damaged or malfunctioning heart valves or for stints to be implanted to open constricted arteries.

Rarely, a patient will be recommended for heart transplant if they are determined to be an approved candidate for one, meaning they are otherwise healthy, so that their body will not reject the replaced organ.

What Do We Know about Asthma?

In many cases, the prognosis for CHF can be good with proper treatment and with close monitoring of treated patients by a qualified MD or cardiologist.

Why is my Asthma Aggravated by Laying Flat (Orthopnea)?

I find many medical sources saying GERD is highly associated with asthma and that GERD can cause orthopnea but little on sources in regard to asthma itself (the common garden variety) causing more breathing difficulty when lying flat on ones back. My suspicion is that it's a fairly common thing with asthma and other lung diseases/disorders.

I also feel that anxiety feelings at times, that come from anticipating the chest tightness and constriction of the bronchial tubes which can actually trigger more asthma when one lays flat (at least for those of us with co morbid anxiety) is a contributing factor.

As far as propping up on pillows, I personally find relief doing that if my asthma flares at night.

I can more comfortably lay on my sides or stomach but can still experience a degree of chest tightness in these positions if my asthma is flaring (more-so on my back) but my albuterol inhaler relieves it a great deal, in preparing for a night's sleep.

Additionally, some medical sources state that the same nerve endings affect both the esophagus and lungs and that irritated nerves may send a signal to the lungs to close more, when one takes the supine position as a protection mechanism, to prevent damage to them from any acid that seeps into the windpipe. The lungs in-essence develop learned behaviors after repeated exposure to small amounts of stomach acid as kind of a self-preservation reaction.

Most sources that refer to the "supine" position, describe it as "lying flat" but I personally used to think that both sitting and lying down placed one in varied supine positions. I thought standing up was the only non-supine position but apparently you have to be lying flat for it to meet the "supine" definition.

What Does Chest and Arm Pain with Difficulty Breathing Indicate?

I would be very concerned if I experienced that set of symptoms together because that could indicate the onset of a heart attack. I would handle it by going to a hospital ER because if it is heart-related, they can administer treatment, to prevent further heart damage and possibly save a person's life. Typical asthma does not usually present with body pain, other than mild chest pain and discomfort and occasional headaches.

On the other hand, those symptoms can also indicate something benign, such as a panic attack or a severe episode of acid reflux but, unless a person knows this, following an initial attack, they would not know that it wasn't their heart, so should seek emergency care ASAP. If chronic anxiety is diagnosed, they could then simply deal with further attacks with anti-anxiety medication and/or anxiety coping methods, such as relaxation techniques, slowed deep breathing from the diaphragm, and diversion methods (things that draw attention away from anxiety symptoms).

Conclusion:

When any of the symptoms of respiratory dysfunction are experienced, as described in the preceding chapters, it is very important to see a qualified medical professional for further evaluation, as soon as possible. The earlier that conditions of asthma and COPD can be diagnosed and treated, the better chances are of symptom-control and prevention of further lung damage.

(END)

www.ingramcontent.com/pod-product-compliance
Lightning Source LLC
Chambersburg PA
CBHW050346290526
45785CB00006B/2653